Office and Home Tai Chi

Tai Chi

AUTHENTIC TAI CHI YOU CAN PRACTICE
ANYWHERE FOR GOOD HEALTH AND IMMUNITY

Yue Zhang

REAL DEAL PRESS
Orlando Florida

Original Chinese Edition of Office & Home Tai Chi by Zhang Yue Published by Shandong Pictorial Publishing House, Shandong Province, P.R. China. All Rights Reserved

Translation, Editing, Book Design and Graphics English edition by James R Martin   Cover Art Work by Yishan Cheng

Publisher's Cataloging-in-Publication

Zhang, Yue

Office and Home Tai Chi: Authentic Tai Chi You Can Practice Anywhere For Good Health and Immunity 1st English edition.
         p.cm.

ISBN-13: 978-0-9827023-9-0

Physical Fitness

Health

Tai Chi

Psychology - Mindfulness

Medical Advice Disclaimer
DISCLAIMER: THIS BOOK DOES NOT PROVIDE MEDICAL ADVICE

The information, including but not limited to, text, graphics, images and other material contained in this book are for informational purposes only. No material in this book is intended to be a substitute for professional medical advice, diagnosis or treatment. Always seek the advice of your physician or other qualified health care provider with any questions you may have regarding a medical condition or treatment and before undertaking a new health care regimen, and never disregard professional medical advice or delay in seeking it because of something you have read in this book.

Table of Contents

About the Author

Born in Shandong China, Yue Zhang holds a master's degree from Shandong Normal University. He majored in Physical Education as an undergraduate and Native Traditional Sports as a graduate student. He has excellent abilities in Kung Fu, Tai Chi and traditional healthcare technologies. He has written about and done research into the application and training of attacking skills of Wushu Sanda for the Journal of Wushu in 2011. He wrote the Introduction to Fan Zi Quan, Journal of Martial Arts in 2014 and wrote Home TAI CHI for Shandong Pictorial Publishing House in 2020. Since July 2007 he has taught at The Institute of Physical Education, University of Jinan where he also does research about Chinese Kung Fu and traditional Chinese health care technologies. From September 2013 to September 2014 he taught Tai Chi and Moving Meditation at The University of Arizona.

Zhang Yue is a member of The USA Wushu-Kungfu Federation (USAWKF). Holder of 6th Duan (grade 6 certificate, the highest professional rank issued by the Chinese Wushu Association[CWA]. He has achieved the Tai Chi First Place at 2017 Golden State International Wushu Championships and the Xing Yi First Place at 2017 Golden State International Wushu Championships. He was Chief Editor of Education Volume of The New Encyclopedia of Chinese Culture.

Acknowledgments

Thank you Mr. Yi-Yuan Lee, coach of the national US Wushu Sanshou Team as a consultant for this book

Appreciation to Xu Yi (Yeats Hsu) for his efforts in getting the English edition published in the United States.

Preface

Office and Home Tai Chi includes two parts, *Limber Up Exercise* and *Xing Qi Tai Chi - Moving Meditation Exercise*. It is a combination of physical exercise and therapy for modern people to keep fit in the office or at home. *Office and Home Tai Chi* is based on ancient Chinese theories of health care including the running laws of blood, Qi (氣)- Vital Energy Flow and Jing Luo (經絡) system-Meridian and Collateral Channels.

Office and Home Tai Chi has presented these ideas in the US since 2013 in a form adapted for westerners to understand and practice when space and time are limited. *Office and Home Tai Chi* helps people work out effectively in an office or at home to improve their health and immunity as an indoor exercise everyday. It may also be useful in case of a public health emergency or crisis when travel is limited.

It is well known that Tai Chi has great health benefits as an important part of Chinese Kung Fu. However, the lengthy traditional Tai Chi routines are complicated and limited by space and time for most individuals. People have to spend a lot of time remembering movements and understanding the true meaning. So, it is less suitable for busy groups of young and middle-aged people. The tedious routine and the culture differences have become the biggest obstacles for Westerner to learn Tai Chi.

Office and Home Tai Chi has removed tedious movements and kept the most important and worthiest elements. Furthermore, it incorporates Tu Na (吐納)- Breathing Exercises and Moving Meditation strengthening the muscles and bones, even nourishing the viscera (various organs in the body).

Office & Home Tai Chi is a concise and efficient regimen. Just twelve minutes of exercise in the office or living room is enough to ease fatigue and promote body function and potential.

Immunity to virus and working efficiency will be naturally improved as well. Businesses encouraging their staffs to practice *Office and Home Tai Chi* before work or during coffee break is not only a benefit, it is also an investment in terms of productivity of the business in the long run!

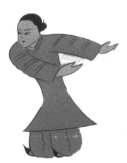

Please Note

All "Figure" illustrations found in this book are mirror images.

Left is to your left, Right is to your right.

Office & Home Tai Chi

INTRODUCTION TO THE METHOD AND HOW IT WORKS

A good immune system is closely related to a better body constitution. Office and Home Tai Chi incorporates different essential elements of Kung Fu, Tai Chi and breathing exercises to keep people fit. It is based on the Traditional Chinese Medicine theory that Qi (氣)- Vital Energy Flow and blood are correlated by Jing Luo (經絡) - Meridian and Collateral Channels.

Office and Home Tai Chi includes two parts: *Limber Up Exercises and Xing Qi Tai Chi - Moving Meditation Exercise.* The motions of Limber Up Exercise are mainly in line with The Twelve Vital Meridians (Shi Er Jing Mai) which are the main stems of Jing Luo system connecting the organs and skin as a whole cycle through which Qi (氣)- Vital Energy Flow circulates around the body.

As the Chinese saying goes, "If your body feels pain, it means your Meridian and Collateral Channels are blocked."

Conversely one will feel good, if Qi -(氣)- Vital Life Energy Flow in the body moves smoothly through the Meridian and Collateral Channels. With the help of proper breath and meditation methods, Meridian and Collateral Channels will be fully opened so that the blood and energy circulation can be enhanced as well.

Office and Home Tai Chi was first introduced and promoted in the United States in 2013. The author found that traditional Tai Chi routines were too complicated and limited by space and time. A lot of time is spent trying to remember intricate moves and remember their meaning. Because of this, traditional methods of practicing Tai Chi are difficult for busy young and middle-aged people to learn. The tedious routine and the cultural differences are the biggest obstacles for Westerners to learn Tai Chi.

While keeping essential parts of traditional Tai Chi, the author incorporated additional essentials of Kung Fu and Chi Gong in *Office and Home Tai Chi* to make it suitable for people from different areas and cultural backgrounds of the world. It is convenient to practice these exercises in the office or at home.

Office and Home Tai Chi has been popularized among different universities, companies and communities in the U.S. including The University of Arizona, Castillo and Associates Insurance Company and others. In 2014, the author cooperated with Mel & Enid Zuckerman College of Public Health, University of Arizona to research the effect and mechanism of Xing Qi (星期) Tai Chi - Moving Meditation Exercise while it was promoted on the campus. They found it had positive results.

Xing Qi (星期) Tai Chi - Moving Meditation Exercise has proved to be effective for improving body function and immunity,

2

especially good for those with health issues. For more fruitful results long-term workouts are necessary. Consistent practice may help prevent some common diseases such as spondylosis, shoulder periarthritis, arthritis, hypertension and neurasthenia etc.

Office and Home Tai Chi consists of Limber Up Exercises and Xing Qi Tai Chi - Moving Meditation Exercises. Each area has special affects and requirements. They can be practiced as a whole or separately according to time and location conditions. It is advised to practice the Limber Up Exercise and the Xing Qi Tai Chi at least one time per day.

Breathing practices recommended in this book are derived from Tu Na a very important part of Qigong 氣功. Breathing influences the well-being of the body, emotional health, and promotes oxygen circulating in the blood. Qigong practices can balance and harmonize the circulation Qi (vital life energy} in the body.

All exercises include breathing along with movements. The exercises are simple in appearance but the basis for their effectiveness is defined by moving the Qi (氣) internally. If you do the exercises regularly and as described you will increase the flow of Qi (氣) or vital life energy throughout your body. This in turn attracts external Qi (氣) to the flow.

Meditation is part of the exercises. In this context meditation is being mindful of what you are doing with the practice and the movements externally and internally. Stay present. Your only thoughts should be feeling the flow and the movement of your body and Qi. In this way you will begin to feel the flow of Qi (星期)vital energy) as you do the exercise. Being mindful, meditating means being there with the flow of the exercise.

The Meridian System

Traditional Chinese Medicine believes the body consists of a network of channels known as the meridian system. This web of paths links together different parts of the body and organs.

Traditional Chinese Medicine created a map of these routes through which Qi - 星期 (vital life energy) flows to every part of the body. This flow of Qi energy helps blood flow and maintains the balance of Yin and Yang. It also increases immunity against illness and disease.

Acupuncture Points

Along these channels are acupuncture points. These are junctions, places through which the qi of the organs and meridians is transported to the body surface. It is generally believed that diseases can be treated when the affected meridians or the affected organs are cleared. Acupuncturists work on these points to regulate corresponding organs or meridians so that the body can return to a state of balance and health.

Twelve Meridians

The system is composed of the twelve regular meridians which form the major structure; they in turn branch out to twelve large collaterals that enter the chest, abdomen and head connecting the internal organs (see Chapter 4).

There are also twelve small collaterals for controlling the muscles and tendons, and smaller collaterals distributed on the skin surface, and the eight extra meridians to enhance the communications and functions within the system.

All the channels work closely with each other. A dysfunction in one path can affect another. In Traditional Chinese Medicine, knowledge of the meridian system is as vital as anatomy and physiology are in Western medicine.

Chapter 4 of this book shows a collection of drawings that will help you understand the twelve meridians and their connections through out the body. All of the exercises take into account the twelve meridians.

Meridians may become blocked. This will result in everything from discomfort and inflammation to disease. The basis for Chinese Acupuncture is to relieve the blockages. In the same way these Tai Chi exercises and self-massage techniques may also relieve pain and eliminate blockages in the system. Self-massage techniques are explained in Chapter 4.

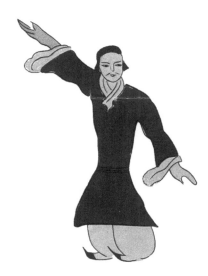

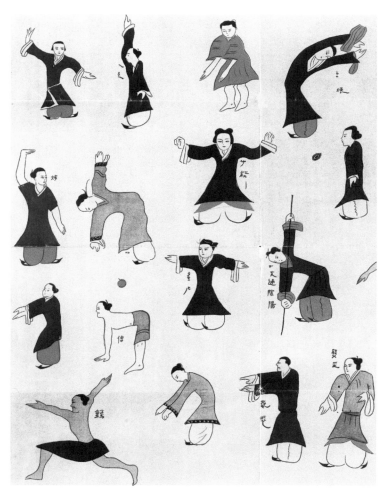

Based on the physical exercise chart; a painting on silk depicting the practice of Qigong Taiji; unearthed in 1973 in Hunan Province, China, from the 2nd-century BC Western Han burial site of Mawangdui Han tombs site, Tomb Number 3.

CHAPTER 2

LIMBER UP EXERCISES

The main purpose of the Limber Up Exercises are to strengthen and smooth *The Twelve Meridian Tendons, Shí èr Jīng* - (十二經筋) by five sets of stretching exercises.

The Twelve Meridian Tendons are made up of muscles and ligaments that reinforce the joints and bones to maintain normal movement function. The joints and bones are nourished by the twelve channels of vital meridians TCM (shí èr jīng mài (十二經脈) -that are symmetrically located on both sides of the body.

However, the directions of the-Twelve Meridian Tendons are in line with Twelve Vital Meridians. Limber Up Exercises are a special way to open the Meridian and Collateral Channels for expelling toxin out of the body to make the body balanced.

In addition to Tai Chi, there are some other traditional Chinese fitness exercises such as Five Animal Exercise (Wu Qin Xi - 五禽戲), Eight Brocade Exercise (Ba Duan Jin - 八段錦), the Tendon-Change Exercise and others. The common characteristic shared by all of them is their slow and soft motions for turning the body and stretching the limbs.

7

Limber Up Exercises are a combination of fitness exercises and self-massage. Along with the movements, we massage the body according to the distribution of Meridian Tendons and Meridians to achieve a physical therapy effect. There is no special requirements of breath and meditation for the Limber Up Exercises. They can be looked at as independent exercises or warming up exercises that are done before doing Xing Qi Tai Chi.

SECTION I   TURTLE TIGER STYLE

1. Be relaxed and stand with your feet together. Allow your arms to hang naturally at your sides, with body upright and eyes looking forward (Figure 1).

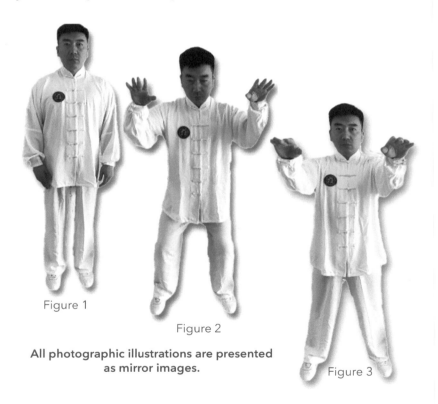

Figure 1

Figure 2

All photographic illustrations are presented as mirror images.

Figure 3

2. Bend the knees and relax the hips slightly. Take the left foot to the left moving feet apart at shoulder width. Raise the arms slowly to eye height with elbows down (Figure 2 page 8).

Continuing the last movement, move the arms back and lower your body. At the same time, stretch the neck forward and sink the lower back making the hips move backward
(Figure 3 page 8 and Figure 4 below).

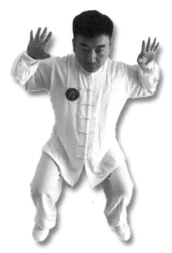

Figure 4

3. Continuing the last movement, bend back your neck when your hands are close to the ears and stand up slowly. Bring the elbows down and push the hands out with palms facing forward (Figures 4 and 5).

This movement imitates the characteristics of turtle making the body move like a wave. *Repeat moves 1 through 5 seven times*.

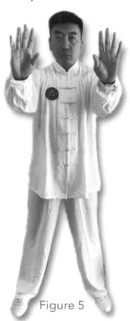

Figure 5

Repeat 1 thru 5 x 7.

4. After finishing the seventh turtle style movement, bend your knees slightly, sink the body and move your hands down placing them on both sides of your navel (Figure 6).

Then straighten up and raise your hands, palms in to nipple height with the inner sides of the wrists clinging to the body (Figure 7).

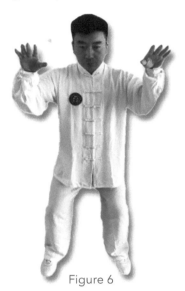

Figure 6

Bend knees, move hands down level with navel.

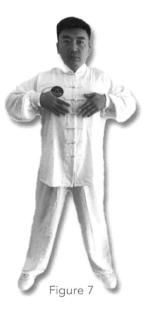

Figure 7

Straighten legs and move hands mid-chest.

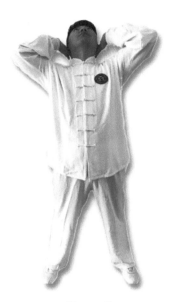

Figure 8

5. Continuing the last movement, bend the body back slowly with legs straight to shape a slight inverse arch of your back. At the same time, raise your hands upward to make them massage your neck and then the back of your head (Figure 8).

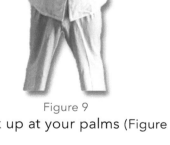

Figure 9

Next, raise your hands over your head fully stretching your arms. Look up at your palms (Figure 9).

6. Bend your body forward and downward almost horizontal with outstretched   arms lowered to shoulder height. Keep your legs straight and look forward. At the same time, flex the fingers making the shape of tiger claw (Figure 10).

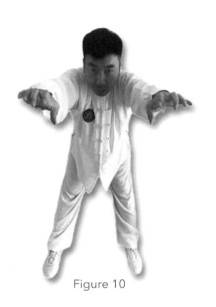

Figure 10

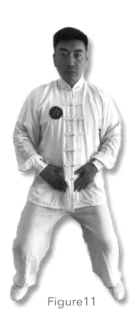

Figure11

7. Bend the knees with the body rising up and take back the hands placing them on both sides of the navel. You are imitating the movement characteristics of a preying tiger and making the body move like waves (Figure 11).

8. And so on, repeat above motions 1 - 7 seven times.

TURTLE TIGER STYLE ACTION TIPS

1. Try to make your hips move in line with your legs when you bend your body to imitate the motion of a tiger preying. Do not allow your hips to move back.

2. Try to relax the whole body and make the movements like waves.

FUNCTIONS

1. Excise the shoulders and spin to ease neck discomfort and prevent shoulder periarthritis and cervical spondylosis.

2. Stretch the muscles and ligaments of the torso and leg

3. *Coordinate Ren Meridian and Du Meridian -*

All of the Office Home Tai Chi exercises take into account the Twelve Vital Meridians of which the Ren and Du Meridians are important.

REN MERIDIAN - CONCEPTION VESSEL

Ren Meridian - Conception Vessel arises from the lower belly, goes up through the center line of trunk to the jaw where it divides into two branches along the both sides of the nose up to the inferior orbit.

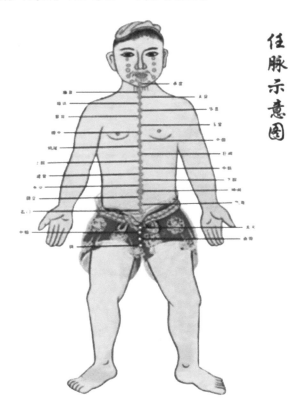

Ren Meridian governs all the meridians of Yin - Former Feminine Principle. Regulating it and its main acupuncture points are good for healing and preventing impotence, premature ejaculation, nocturnal emission, menstrual colic, gastritis, abdominal distension, chest ache, chest congestion, convulsion, and vomiting.

See Chapter 4 (appendices) for full details and additional information on the functions of each of the Twelve Vital Meridians - Shi Er Jing Jin (十二經筋).

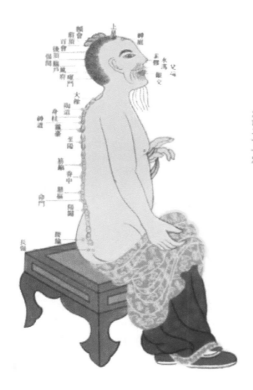

督脈之圖

穴計二十七穴 已上本經中行幕

Du Meridian - Governor Vessel arises from the lower belly going down through the perineum and then perineum and then goes up along the spine all the way to the top of the head - Bai Hui acupuncture point. It governs all the meridians of Yang - Former Masculine Principle

DU MERIDIAN - GOVERNOR VESSEL

Conception Vessel and Governor Vessel in order to balance Yin (Feminine energy) and Yang (Masculine energy) - two opposite energies in the human body.

Increases positive energy and strength. It also has the function of stimulating Leg Greater Yin Kidney Meridian.

Regulating Du Meridian and its main acupuncture points are good for healing and preventing back problems, infant convulsion, headache, dizziness and the male disease such as kidney deficiency and impotence etc.

SECTION 2 APE STYLE

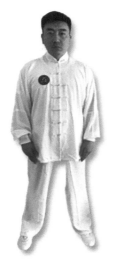

1. Stand naturally with feet apart at shoulder width and arms hanging alongside the body (Figure 12).

2. Raise your hands above your head from both sides of the body with the palms facing forward. Grab the right hand with the left hand and pull slightly making the upper body bend to the left at about 30 degrees (Figure 13 and 14).

Figure 12

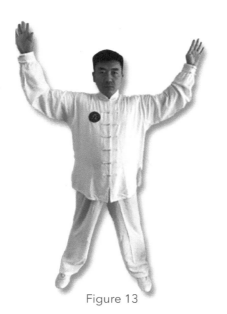

Figure 13

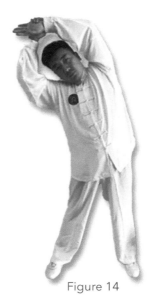

Figure 14

16

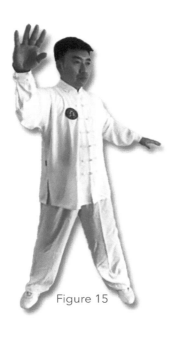

Figure 15

3. After bending for two seconds, turn your body slightly to the right and return upright.

Simultaneously, arms swing to the right. The left hand moves above the right shoulder to flap its back for two times.

At the same time, the right hand swings all the way back to gently massage the Shen Yu Acupuncture point of the right lower back two times with the back of the hand.

Shen Yu Acupuncture points are located on both sides of the spine symmetrically. Each of them is about 1.5 inches to the second lumbar spinous process adjacent (Figure 15 and 16).

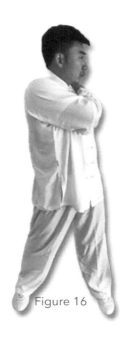

Figure 16

17

4. Return to the original position by turning your body turn to the left from position in figure 16 to figure 17. After pausing a little bit, do the same motion in the opposite direction.

Repeat series 12 - 17 three times.

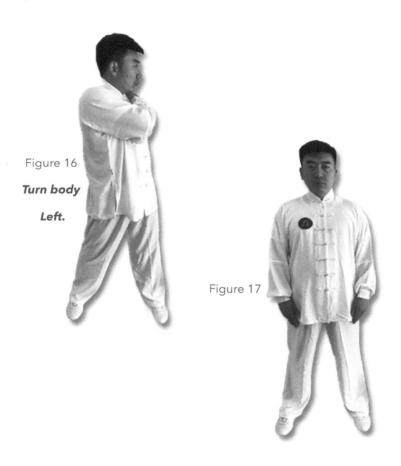

Figure 16

Turn body

Left.

Figure 17

APE STYLE ACTION TIPS

1. Keep the hips upright when bending the trunk.

2. Turning the body to bring the arms and hands in place for massaging the shoulder and lower back.

FUNCTIONS

1. Stretch both sides of the torso and the shoulders.

 2. Coordinate *Arm Lesser Yin Heart Meridian (page 71)* and *Arm Greater Yang Small Intestine Meridian (page 77)* that aid in the activities of boosting heart function and promoting digestion and absorption.

SECTION 3: ARCHERY STYLE

1. Stand up with feet apart at shoulder width. Arms hanging naturally at your sides (Figure 18).

2. Raise your left arm laterally with five fingers up straight while raising the right forearm to the upper left to put your right fist on the left side of your chest (Figure 19).

3. The left arm swings to the right side of the body horizontally. Meanwhile, the right fist turns into palm with the thumb points up to stroke the inner side of the left arm from the left chest all the way to the palm until the two palms get put together at the right side of the body. The body should turn right following above motion (Figures 20 and 21).

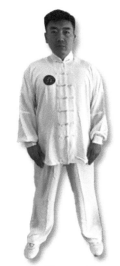

Figure 18

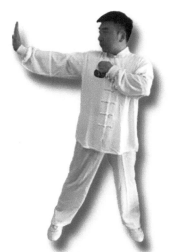

Figure 19

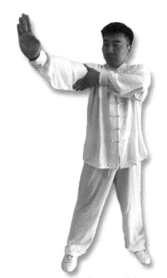

Figure 20

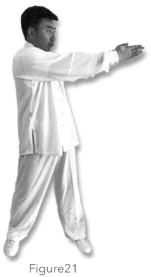

Figure21

4. The left arm swings to the left horizontally. Following along with the left arm, the right-hand twists inward to put on the back of the left palm to stroke outer side of the left arm all the way to the back of the left shoulder (Figures 22 and 23).

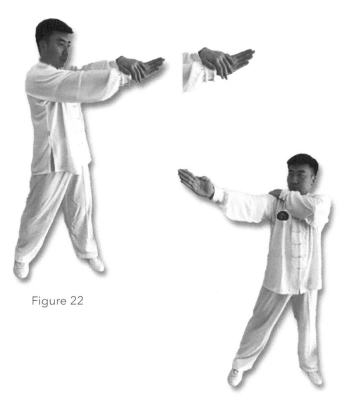

Figure 22

Figure 23

22

5. Continuing the last movement, your left arm swings back to left side of the body and you put the right palm on the back of your neck by raising the right forearm over your head (Figure 24).

6. Your right hand strokes your neck to the right horizontally while your head turns right with eyes looking toward right hand (Figure 25).

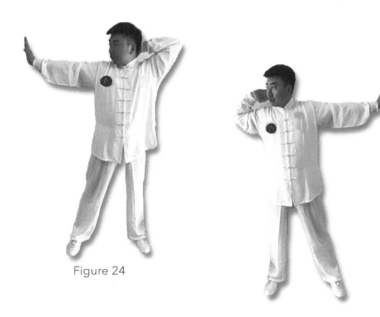

Figure 24

Figure25

7. Continuing the last movement, the right arm stretches out from shoulder level. At the same time, the fingers of each hand keep closed and point up. Head returns with your eyes looking forward (Figure 26).

8. Arms down return to the original position (Figure 27).

9. Repeat above motions in the opposite direction.

10. Repeat entire ten moves three times in each direction.

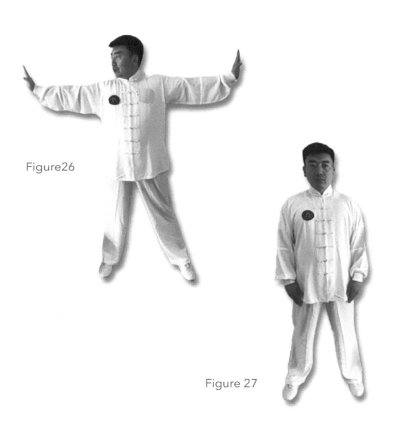

Figure26

Figure 27

ACTION TIPS

1. Your hand should stay on the arm slightly when while you stroke it.

2. When you swing your arms, your body should turn with it.

FUNCTIONS

1. Conditions the neck and the shoulders.

2. Coordinates *Arm Brightness Yang Large Intestine Meridian (page 68), Arm Lesser Yang Triple Burner Meridian (page 84), Arm Greater Yin Lung Meridian (page 66), and Arm Absolute Yin Pericardium Meridian (page 82)*. It may relive throat inflammation, clear the lungs and refresh ourselves.

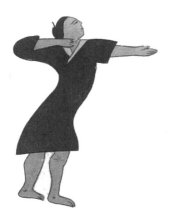

See Chapter 4 for diagrams and drawings tracing each of the twelve meridians.

SECTION 4: ARHAT STYLE

1. Relax and stand up with feet apart at shoulder width with arms hanging at sides naturally (Figure28).

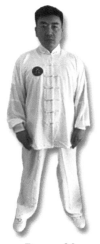

Figure 28

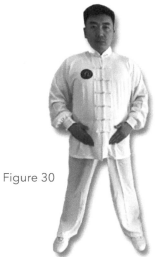

Figure
29

2. Raise your hands, palms to the head with the middle fingers put on both corners of the forehead. Move your palms move down to stroke your face, then your neck and all the way down to the top of your thighs down the body (Figure 29 and 30).

Figure 30

26

3. Continuing the last movement, bend the upper body down and stroke the front sides of your legs with the palms of your hands down to the tip of your toes keeping your legs straight, if possible. (Figure 31)

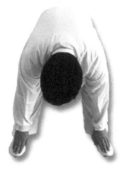

Figure 31

4. Move your hands from the tip of your toes to the insides of the ankles to stroke the insides of both legs all the way up to the chest along the body, rising up gradually following the motion (Figures 32 and 33).

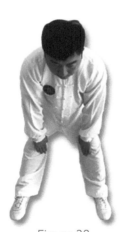

Figure 32

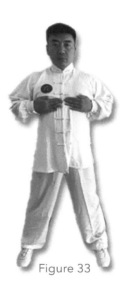

Figure 33

27

5. Move your palms to your back and stroke your body down to the hips. Continuing the last movement, stroke the backs of both legs with your palms all the way to the ankles with the upper body gradually bending down (Figures 34, 35 and 36).

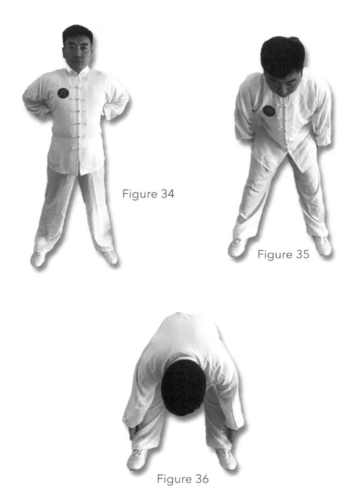

Figure 34

Figure 35

Figure 36

6.Move your palms around your insteps to the insides of the ankles to stroke up the insides of both legs to the thigh and lower body rising up gradually following the motion. Continue the last movement, moving your palms stroke over groin, returning to the original position. (Figures 37, 38 and 39)

7. Repeat the above series of movements three times.

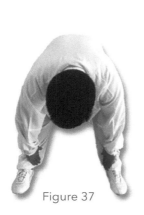

Figure 37

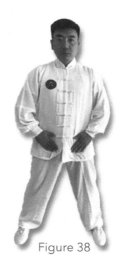

Figure 38

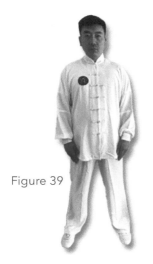

Figure 39

ACTION TIPS

1. Try to keep legs straight when stroking or patting the insides and backs of both legs.

FUNCTIONS

1. Extend upward and massage the muscles and ligaments of your torso and legs.

2. Coordinating *Leg Brightest Yang Stomach Meridian (77), Leg Last Yin Liver Meridian (88), and Leg Greater Yin Spleen Meridian (74).* This has the function of aiding digestion, improving eyesight and easing mental stress.

SECTION 5: PHOENIX STYLE

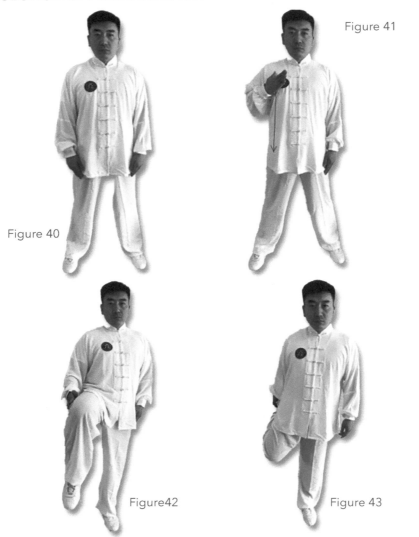

Figure 41

Figure 40

Figure42

Figure 43

1. Stand with feet apart at shoulder width. Arms hanging naturally with the hands, palms in on the outer sides of the legs, your eyes looking forward (Figure 40).

2. Using the palm of the left hand rise up to the outer side of the chest then stroke the body down to the waist (Figure 41).

3. Continuing the last movement, shift the weight onto the right foot. Raise the left knee and stroke the outer side of the leg with the left hand until you grab the tips of your toes to pull the leg back (Figures 42 and 43).

4. Raise your right arm to shoulder height with fingers pointing forward together. The body is shaped like a bow from side view. Try to keep facing forward (Figure 44).

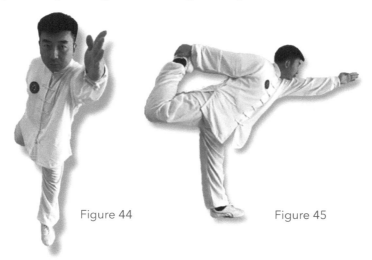

Figure 44   Figure 45

5. Continuing the last movement, extend the left leg slightly leaning the body forward so that you extend the left side of the body and the front part of left leg.
Stop pulling when you feel your back tense slightly. Release the left foot making the leg stretch back with toes pointed. At the same time, the left arm stretches out backwards at shoulder height with fingers pointing forward together. Meanwhile, the whole body is stretched with the limbs be straight and keeping balance (Figure 45).

31

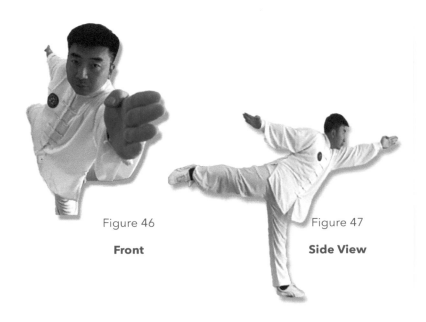

Figure 46

Front

Figure 47

Side View

6. Keeping your weight on the right foot, raise the upper body. Meanwhile, move the left leg and left arm back (Figure 46 and 47 side view).

7. Then return to the original position (Figure 48 and 49).

8. Repeat above movements (1 - 7) in the opposite direction.

9. Repeat the entire series of motions three times.

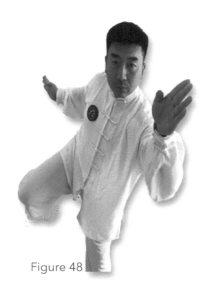

Figure 48

**Returning to
standing position**

Demonstration video at:
JRMartinMedia.com
-Real Deal Press - Office
and Home Tai Chi

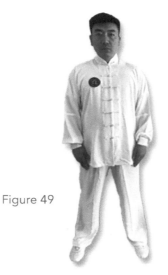

Figure 49

ACTION TIPS

1. The difficulty of this section is keeping your balance. If the body leans to one side, turning the front arm to the other side slightly is a good way to regulate the weight center for keeping your balance.

2. When the body is shaped like a bow, there will be a counter force between the bent leg and the grabbing arm. Be sure not to extend the leg too hard for the sake of safety. Stop extending as soon as your back gets tight.

FUNCTIONS

1. Extends the muscles of the back and the front part of the legs.

2. Coordinate *Leg Lesser Yang Gallbladder Meridian (page 86), Leg Greater Yang Bladder Meridian (page 78), and Leg Brightest Yang Stomach Meridian (page 72)* in order to prevent and relieve headache and cervical pain. It also has the diuretic and digestive function.

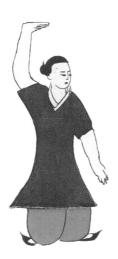

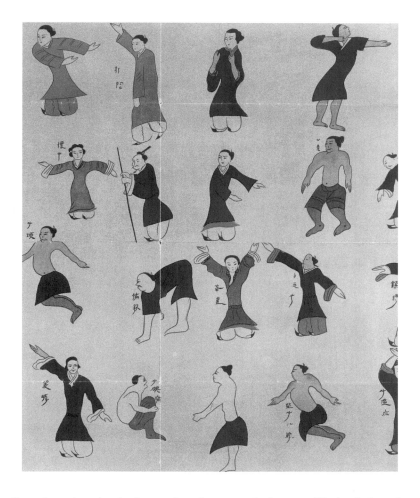

Based on the physical exercise chart; a painting on silk depicting the practice of Qigong Taiji; unearthed in 1973 in Hunan Province, China, from the 2nd-century BC Western Han burial site of Mawangdui Han tombs site, Tomb Number 3.

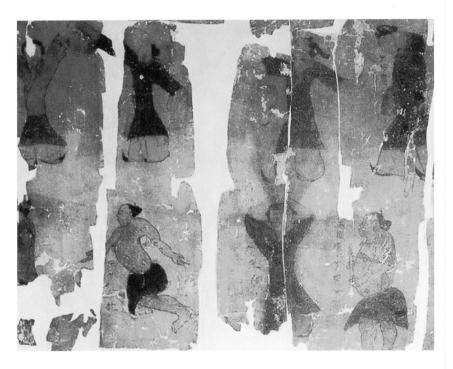

The original physical exercise chart; a painting on silk depicting the practice of Qigong Taiji; unearthed in 1973 in Hunan Province, China, from the 2nd-century BC Western Han burial site of Mawangdui Han tombs site, Tomb Number 3.

XING QI TAI CHI MOVING MEDITATION EXERCISE

Xing Qi Tai Chi - Moving Meditation originated from the ancient Chinese Tiao Xi Gong (調息功). *Moving Meditation. Xing Qi Tai Chi is different from the Limber Up Exercise. Its motions should be coordinated with proper breathing and guided spiritually.*

The main purpose of *Xing Qi Tai Chi* is to motivate potential energy, which means enhancing the flow of Qi (氣) and making them circulate all around the body for improving the vitality.

Regular practice of *Xing Qi Tai Chi* is a strategy to help people maintain young and healthy lives. From a western medicine point of view, it can improve the central nervous system excitability, promote blood circulation and relax the muscles through mental activity regulation, breath control and posture adjustment.

Practicing *Xing Qi Tai Chi* helps coordinate abdominal breathing helping the diaphragm move with breathing. Expanding the belly by inhaling deeply will make the diaphragm sink to push organs downward. As a result, the diaphragm goes up more than usual while exhaling which could help expel more carbon dioxide that may be left at the bottom of the lungs.

For the best effect, it is better to practice Xing Qi Tai Chi before exercising or working in the morning. Be sure not to practice in the evening before going to bed, because it may result in sleeplessness because of over excitement.

READY POSITION

1. Be relaxed and stand straight with feet together. *Look forward and close your lips lightly with the tip of your tongue touching the roof of your mouth.* Arms should be hanging naturally (Figure 1).

2. Relax. Try to eliminate all the distractions in your mind. Breathe gently but deeply through your nose to the abdomen. Allow you abdomen to rise as it fills with air. Exhale from the abdomen back out your nose. As you meditate on your breath allow it to be as natural as possible moving through nose to abdomen and back..

3. Bend the knees and relax the hips slightly. Raise your left heel as you take a half step to the left and breathe in. Begin to breathe out as soon as the left foot touches the ground placing feet apart at shoulder width (Figure 2).

Xing Qi Tai Chi Moving Meditation Exercise Demonstration

Go to jrmartinmedia.com Real Deal Press for Demo.

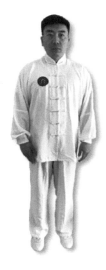

Figure 1

Start with feet together, relax breathe.

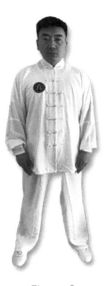

Figure 2 -

Left foot rests shoulder width apart.

2. *SHOULDER CIRCLING*

1. Relax your arms by your sides, move your shoulders forward slightly toward your chest. Then, move your shoulders up with chest expanding as you inhale gradually (Figure 3 and 4)
.

2. Continuing the last movement, move your shoulders back and then down once the chest has been emptied completely. Meanwhile, move both sides of dorsal muscles towards the spin slightly, pulling on your back.

The dorsal muscles of the back in general, including those attaching the shoulder girdle to the trunk posteriorly, the posterior serratus muscles, and the erector spinae. -- Wikipedia

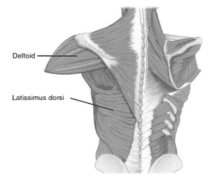

Then relax and return to the ready position. The process should be done while gently exhaling (Figure 5 and 6).

3. Your shoulders will have completed a circular motion through above steps. Repeat the above movements three times with corresponding breathing.

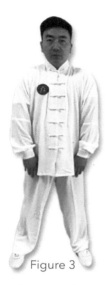

Figure 3

Relax arms, begin
moving shoulders.

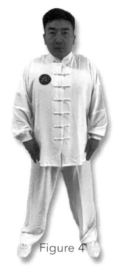

Figure 4

Shoulders move up,
inhale as chest expands
gradually.

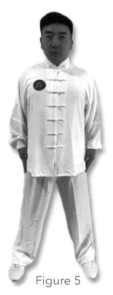

Figure 5

Shoulders move back
and down.

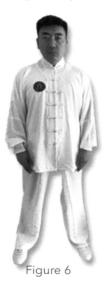

Figure 6

Move dorsal muscles
while exhaling then relax.

3. PUSH MOUNTAIN

1. Slowly raise the arms forward with palms facing down and inhale. Turn the palms upright slowly until they reach the shoulder level with fingers separated slightly and begin to exhale.

At the same time, meditate that Qi (氣) - Vital Energy Air goes simultaneously from the tips of the thumbs of both hands through the tips of index fingers, middle fingers and ring fingers to the tips of little fingers.

These points on the finger tips are the acupuncture points named Shi Xuan (十宣). Shi Xuan acupuncture points are at the top of each finger about 0.2 mm (1/16th inch) to the edge of the nail (Figures 7 and 8).

2. Move your hands, palms out, back to the front of the chest, relax the shoulders and begin to inhale. Meanwhile, meditate that Lao Gong acupuncture points (勞宮穴) in both palms are opened; through which fresh air from the outside comes into the inner body.

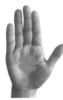

The Lao Gong acupuncture point is at the center of the palms, between the second and third metacarpal bones near to the third one, where the tip of middle finger touches against when you make a fist.

Move your hands, palms out in front of you. Exhale imaging that the air from the bottom of the body is expelled through Lao Gong acupuncture points (Figures 9 and 10.)

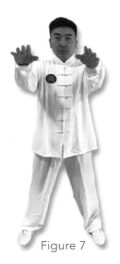

Figure 7

**Raise Arms palms down
breathe in.**

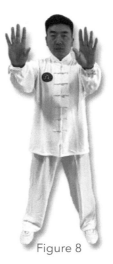

Figure 8

**Hands shoulder level
palms out..**

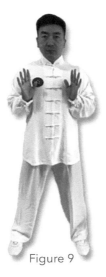

Figure 9

**Move hands palms out
back to front of chest..**

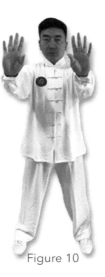

Figure 10

**Move hands, palms out in
front of you.**

4. OPENING AND CLOSING

1. Spread arms apart at shoulder width, hands palms out and then move them back about 30 cm (11.8 inches) toward the shoulders with your elbows down. Inhale during this process (Figures 11 and 12).

2. Turn your hands, palms inward making them face each other. Then bring them close to each other until they are about 20 cm (8 inches) apart.

At the same time, exhale, bend the knees slowly to half squat and concentrate on Lao Gong (勞宮穴) acupuncture points meditating that they are facing each other exactly.
(Figures 13 and 14).

Lao Gong acupuncture points are at the center of the palms. It is where the tip of middle finger touches when you make a fist.

   Lao Gong, is the eighth point of the heart master channel. It is stimulated to ease anxiety and clear inflammation.

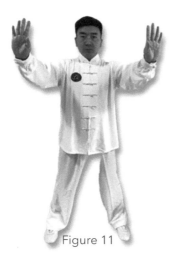

Figure 11

Hold hands up shoulder
height palms out.

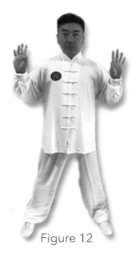

Figure 12

Move arms and hands
back toward shoulders.

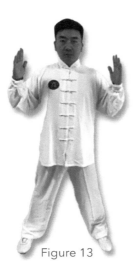

Figure 13

Turn hand in palms
facing each oher..

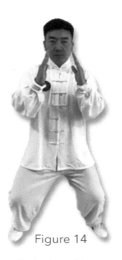

Figure 14

Exhale, bend knees,
move palms to 8" apart..

5. RISING

1. Begin with a half squat, separate your hands to shoulder width and inhale. Then bring your hands, palms facing, close to each other slowly to about 20 cm (8") apart and in tune with breathing while standing up straight.

In the process, exhale and meditate that the Qi (氣) - Vital Energy Air is exchanged between your two palms through Lao Gong (勞宮穴) acupuncture points that are facing each other (Figure 15 and 16).

Lao Gong acupuncture points are at center of the palms. It is where the tip of middle finger touches when you make a fist.

2. Continuing the last movement, raise the heels, move your arms upward and inhale with your eyes following your hands. At the same time, meditate that your fingertips are touching the sky (Figure 3.)

Note: You may be able to feel the Qi (氣) - Vital Energy air flow between your palms from the Lao Gong points in your palms. Meditate on that flow.

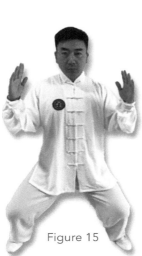

Figure 15

Begin with half squat.

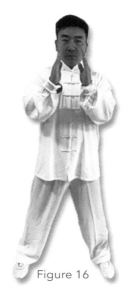

Figure 16

Exhale and stand , feet apart. Hands moving closer together.

Figure 17

Raise the heels of your feet, move arms up, inhale, eyes look up.

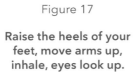

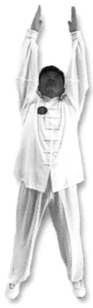

6. LANDING CRANE

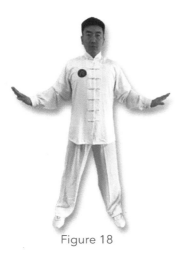

1. Move both arms down laterally to waist height turning your palms outward facing down as you move your arms. Relax the shoulders and move your elbows down. Exhale during this process (Figure 18.)

Figure 18

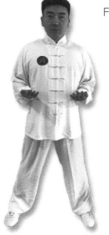

Figure 19

2. Begin to inhale. At the same time turn your palms upward and move them to both sides of your waist (Figure 19).

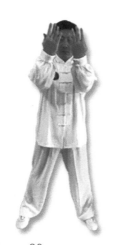

Then move your palms forward and up to make them face to your eyes just like looking into a mirror (Figure 20.

Figure 20

Think of the Lao Gong (勞宮穴) acupuncture points that are now directly in front of your face. Remember the Lao Gong Xue acupuncture points are at center of each palm. It is where the tip of middle finger touches when you make a fist.

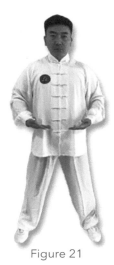

3. Move your hands down in front of your belly with palms facing up (Figure 21).

Figure 21

Then twist your arms inward with your palms facing down. Now draw a circle with, your hands from the inside out to put them down in front of the belly with fingers toward each others. At the same time sink the body slightly. Exhale in this process (Figure 22.)

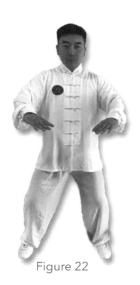

Figure 22

7. MILLING (MOVEMENTS AND ATTENTION FOLLOW HANDS)

1. Shift your weight onto the right foot. Slowly turn your body slightly to the right with your eyes following your hands. Then shift your weight onto left foot while turning the body to left (Figure 23).

Inhale and exhale during this process. Begin to exhale when shifting your weight from foot to foot. (Figure 24). Finally return to face forward as in Figure 25.

2. Do a short pause for a second after returning to the original position (Figure 25), sinking a little bit at the knees while breathing out from the abdominal area.

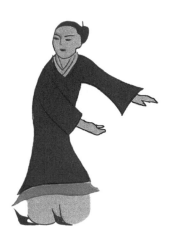

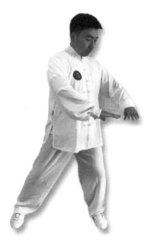

<<Figure 23

Shift weight to right foot,
then turn body to left.
Inhale, exhale.

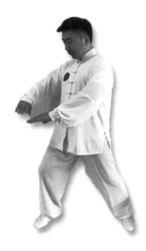

Figure 24 >>

Begin to exhale when
shifting weight..

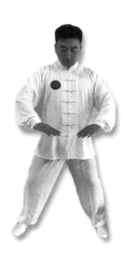

<<Figure 25

Short pause, sink
body, breathe from the
abdominal area.

3. Begin to shift your weight onto left foot and turn your body to left with your eyes following your hands. Then shift the weight onto the right foot slowly and turn the body to right. Inhaling during this process.

Begin exhaling when shifting your weight from one foot to the other foot. Then return your body to face forward. Do a short pause for a second after returning to the original position (Figure 28) sinking a little bit at the knees while breathing out from the abdominal area (Figure 26,27,28).

4. The above symmetrical rotating actions to the left and right are like milling wood in that your attention should follow your hands as you move the object.

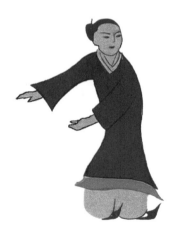

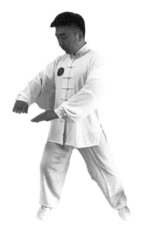

<<Figure 26

**Shift weight to left foot,
then turn body to left.
Inhale, exhale, eyes
follow hands..**

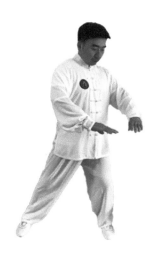

Figure 27>>

**Shift weight to left foot,
then turn body to right.
Inhale, exhale.**

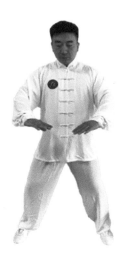

<<Figure 28

**Return to this position.
Knees bent slightly.
Breathe from diaphragm..**

53

8. BENDING BACK

1. Begin by breathing in. Slight crouch. Turn the palms of your hands face up and open the arms laterally (Figure 29).

Straighten up and continue to raise the arms until they are a little higher than the shoulders with the palms facing down (Figure 30).

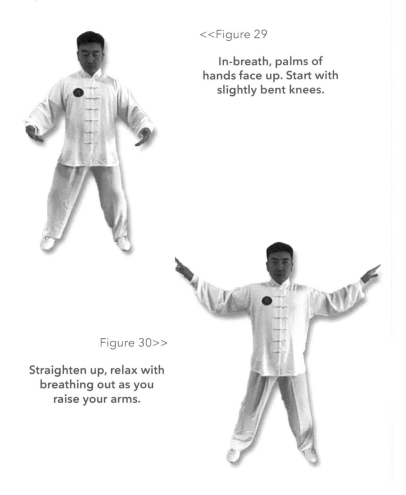

<<Figure 29

In-breath, palms of hands face up. Start with slightly bent knees.

Figure 30>>

Straighten up, relax with breathing out as you raise your arms.

2. Bend your knees at about 45 degree and hold your arms crossed in front of the chest with the right arm outside. Exhale during this process (Figure 31).

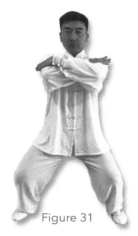

3. Inhale as you straighten up. Stretch your arms out at shoulder height and width. Exhale, as you turn the palms upward and bring them down

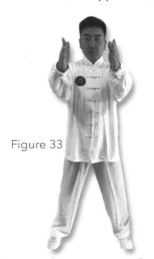

Figure 31

**Bend knees, arms cross
in front of upper chest.**

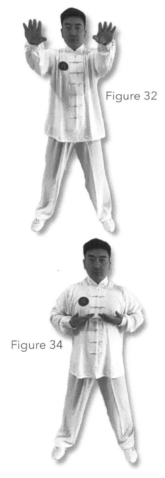

Figure 32

Figure 33

Figure 34

placing the outer sides (little finger in) just below the chest with palms facing up (Figures 32, 33 and 34).

55

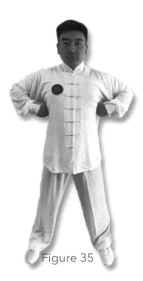

Figure 35

4. As you begin to inhale, turn your palms to make your fingers point back. Then bend the upper body back with the backs of the hands facing downward along both sides of the spine to massage your lower back. Eyes looking up. (Figures 35 and 36, and 37).

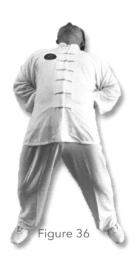

Figure 36

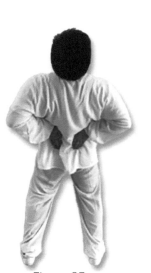

Figure 37
(rear view 36)

Massage with back of hands.

56

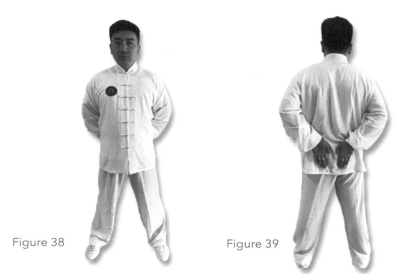

Figure 38   Figure 39

5. Continuing from the last movement, straighten your the body let your hands slide to your hips. (Figures 38 and 39) Then raise the arms laterally to make the fingers cross over the head with palms facing each other and look forward (Figures 40 and 41).

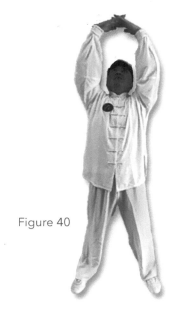

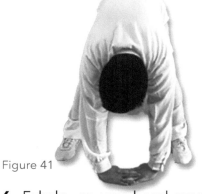

Figure 41

Figure 40

6. Exhale. as you bend your body forward keeping legs straight. Touch palms to touch the ground.

57

9. *RECOVER*

1. Straighten up your body and open your arms like holding a ball, as you gently breathe in (Figure 43).

2. Continue the last movement, overlap your hands on the lower abdomen about 10 cm (4") below your navel which is the position of Dan Tian acupuncture point (丹田穴).

Men should put right hand palm down over the left hand and women the left hand palm down over the right hand. Meditate while breathing in and out from lower abdomen (Figure 44).

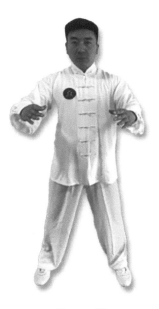 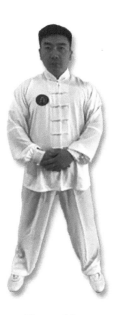

Figure 43   Figure 44

10. BELLY MASSAGE

Use the palms of your hands to massage your belly circularly in counter clockwise direction. This means that your palms move from Dan Tian acupuncture point (丹田穴) to the left side (Figure 45), then up to the pit of the heart, (Figure 46) then to the right side (Figure 47) and return to Dan Tian (丹田) (Figure. 44).

Dan Tian acupuncture point is about 10 cm (4") below the navel. Repeat this three times in counter clockwise direction, then do it in clockwise direction three times. Inhale when the hands move up and exhale when they move down. The power of massage should be in the meditation. Put hands back to both sides of the body after the massage has been finished.

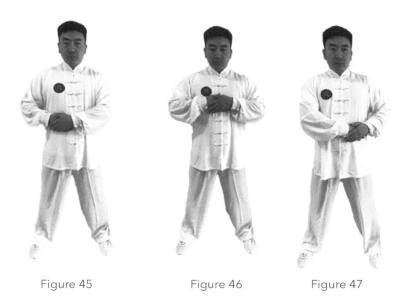

Figure 45   Figure 46   Figure 47

Note: Practice *Xing Qi Tai Chi* for three times continuously every time you do it. After you have finished two times your hands should be put back to both sides of the body before you start again.

When the last cycle is finished, overlap the palms on the lower belly and begin to massage the belly. Rub your hands against each other for forty-nine times to warm them after finishing the belly massage, then put the palms on the face and massage it up and down slightly for nine times.

If you feel numb or inflated in your palms after finishing the exercise, it is called Qi Gan (氣感) . It is the Feel of Vital Energy Air which means good result have been achieved.

Please do not practice before you go to bed, because it will make you sleepless and over excited.

CHAPTER 3 EXERCISE CHART

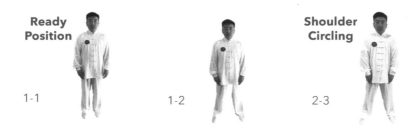

Ready Position

1-1

1-2

Shoulder Circling

2-3

Sections 1 through 10. Pictures listed by section and figure number. Example: Section 3 - Figure 4 -- (3-4)

60

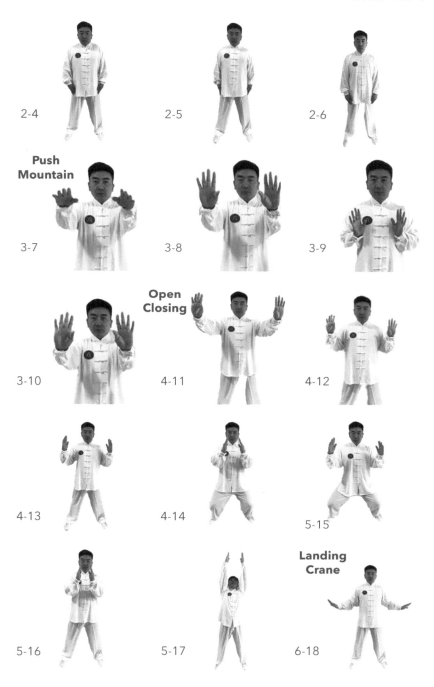

2-4

2-5

2-6

Push Mountain

3-7

3-8

3-9

3-10

Open Closing

4-11

4-12

4-13

4-14

5-15

5-16

5-17

Landing Crane

6-18

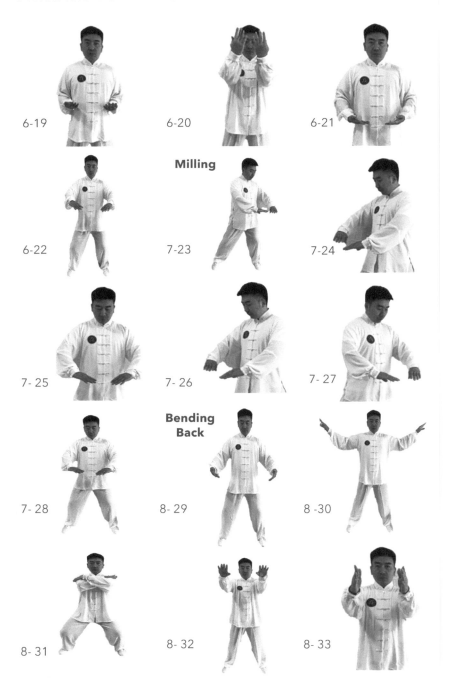

6-19

6-20

6-21

Milling

6-22

7-23

7-24

7- 25

7- 26

7- 27

Bending Back

7- 28

8- 29

8 -30

8- 31

8- 32

8- 33

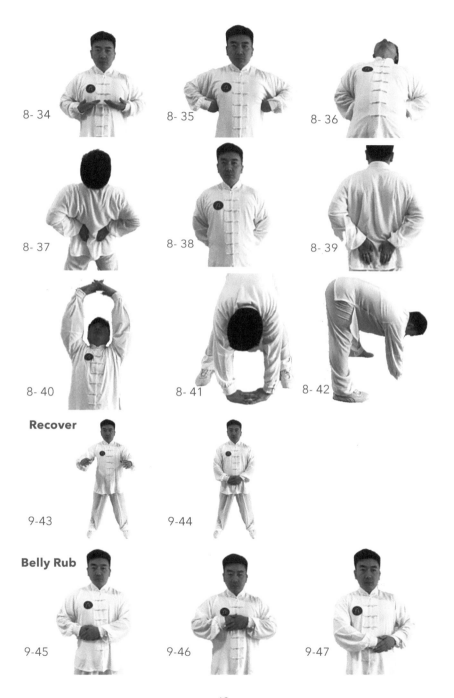

8- 34

8- 35

8- 36

8- 37

8- 38

8- 39

8- 40

8- 41

8- 42

Recover

9-43

9-44

Belly Rub

9-45

9-46

9-47

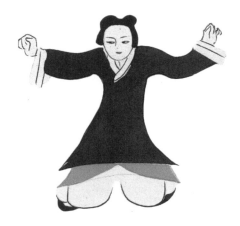

The content in this book is not intended to be a substitute for professional medical advice, diagnosis, or treatment. Always seek the advice of your physician or other qualified health provider with any questions you may have regarding a medical condition.

TWELVE VITAL MERIDIANS - SHI ER JING JIN (十二經筋)

The Functions and Graphs of Twelve Vital Meridians, Ren Meridian (任脈) - Conception Vessel and Du Meridian (督脈) - Governor Vessel

The motions of the *Limber Up Exercise* (Chapter 2) are mainly for stretching or massaging the body in line with Shi Er Jing Jin (十二經筋) -Twelve Meridian Tendons which are in line with Shi Er Jing Mai (十二經脈) - Twelve Vital Meridians.

Twelve Vital Meridians are the main stems of Jing Luo (經絡) system - Meridian and Collateral Channels, which connect the viscera and skin as a whole cycle. So it is necessary to illustrate the directions and functions of Twelve Vital Meridians.

Twelve Vital Meridians are symmetrically located at both sides of the body. The acupuncture points are distributed along these channels.

In addition, *Ren Meridian* (任脈) - *Conception Vessel and Du Meridian* (督脈) - Governor Vessel are respectively on the center line of the front and back of the torso. *Ren Meridian* governs all the meridians of Yin - Former Feminine Principle. *Du Meridian* governs all the meridians of Yang - Former Masculine Principle. Traditional Chinese Medicine holds that all Meridians and Collateral Channels will become fluent if *Ren Meridian and Du Meridian* are unobstructed and connected up. Their trends are presented in the following pictures with brief introduction of its health care functions in the sequence of the flow process.

As for the common person who has no medical specialty, it is an effective self-care practice to relieve illness or discomfort by massaging the limbs or trunk where certain meridians go through and stimulating the corresponding acupuncture points with pressing or kneading methods. (see page)

It is said in Traditional Chinese Medicine (TCM) that proper self massage actions with the hands to relax the muscles and stimulate relevant meridians or acupressure points, will alleviate strain and tiredness. Also prevent and relieve certain illness.

1. ARM GREATER YIN LUNG MERIDIAN (手太陰肺經)

Arm Greater Yin Lung Meridian arises from the abdomen and goes up through the chest to the front shoulder. It then goes along the front inside of the arm all the way to the radialis side of the thumb. Its corresponding organs are the lungs and it is related to the health of the chest, belly, throat and teeth.

Regulating *Arm Greater Yin Lung Meridian* and its main acupuncture points are good for healing and preventing sore throat, cough, asthma, toothache, abdominal distension.

ARM GREATER YIN LUNG MERIDIAN

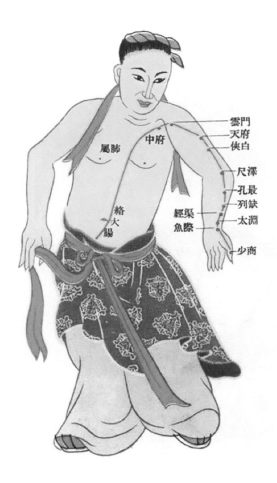

手太陰肺經之圖　凡十一穴　左右共二十二穴

雲門
天府
俠白
尺澤
孔最
列缺
太淵
少商
經渠
魚際
屬肺
中府
絡大腸

67

2. ARM BRIGHTNESS YANG LARGE INTESTINE MERIDIAN (手陽明大腸經)

The Arm Brightness Yang Large Intestine Meridian is connected to the *Arm Greater Yin Lung Meridian.*

It arises from the index finger and goes up through the outer side of the arm, the front shoulder, the neck and the cheek all the way to the side of the nose.

Another branch goes down from the clavicle through the lung and diaphragmatic muscle into the intestine. It is consequential to large intestine and related to the health of the eyes, ears, mouth and lower belly.

Regulating the *Arm Brightness Yang Large Intestine Meridian* and its main acupuncture points are good for healing and preventing tinnitus, hot eyes, stomatitis, facial distortion, lower belly cramp and constipation etc.

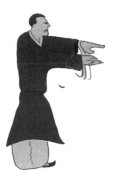

The twelve regular meridians are distributed on both sides of the body symmetrically. Each meridian is paired with corresponding internal organs in groups on the legs, under the arms and yin and yang.

68

ARM BRIGHTNESS YANG LARGE INTESTINE MERIDIAN

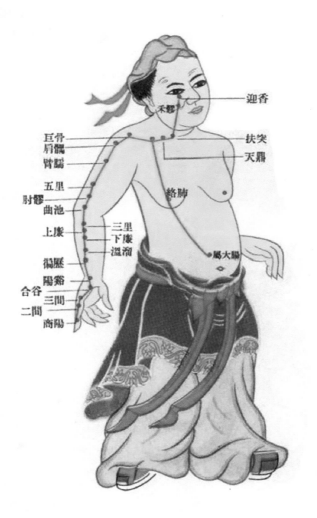

迎香

禾髎

扶突

天鼎

巨骨

肩髃

臂臑

絡肺

五里

肘髎

曲池

三里

下廉

溫溜

上廉

偏歷

陽谿

合谷

三間

二間

商陽

屬大腸

手陽明大腸經之圖

凡二十穴

左右共四十穴

3. ARM LESSER YIN HEART MERIDIAN (手少陰心經)

Arm Lesser Yin Heart Meridian arises from heart with one branch goes down through the diaphragmatic muscle to connect the small intestine. An other branch goes up to the eye with with a branch that goes through the armpit, the back inside of the arm, the palm to the radialis side of little the finger. It is corresponding to heart and related to the health of heart and head.

Regulating the *Arm Lesser Yin Heart Meridian* and its main acupuncture points are good for healing and preventing palpitation, sleeplessness, amnesia and headache etc.

ARM GREATER YIN SPLEEN MERIDIAN

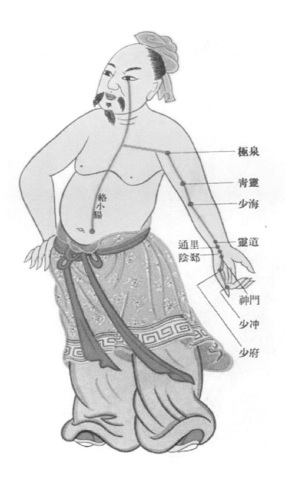

71

LEG BRIGHTNESS YANG STOMACH MERIDIAN

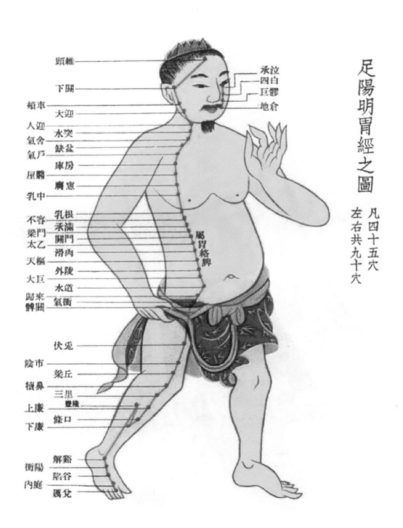

4. *LEG BRIGHTEST YANG STOMACH MERIDIAN*

(足陽明胃經)

Leg Brightest Yang Stomach Meridian arises from the side of the nasal Alar - Ying Xiang acupuncture point (迎香穴) along the nose into the eye and goes up to the forehead. Then it goes down through the front trunk, the front side of the leg and the instep to the inside of the big toe.

Leg Brightest Yang Stomach Meridian is consequential to the stomach and related to the health of the digestive system. Regulating it and its main acupuncture points are good for healing and preventing gastric ulcer, stomach cramp, borborygmus (bowel sound), abdominal pain and diarrhea.

5. *LEG GREATER YIN SPLEEN MERIDIAN* (足太陰脾經)

Leg Greater Yin Spleen Meridian arises from the inside of the big toe and goes up through the inside of the ankle, the shank and the thigh, then goes through the abdomen, the diaphragmatic muscle and the heart and finally into the throat.

It is consequential the to spleen and related to the health of digestive and absorption function.

Regulating the *Leg Greater Yin Spleen Meridian* and its main acupuncture points are good for healing and preventing hemafecia, abdominal distension, abdominal pain, indigestion, inappetence (lack of appetite), backache, weakness, lower limb paralysis, irregular menstruation, nocturnal emission and low sperm.

LEG GREATER YIN SPLEEN MERIDIAN

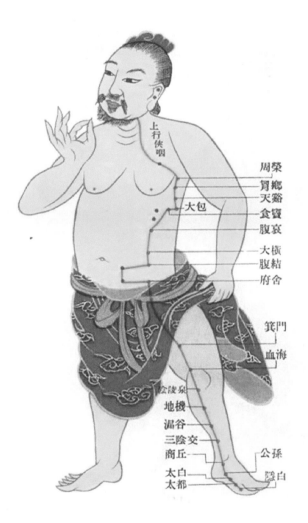

足太陰脾經之圖　凡二十穴　左右共四十穴

上行俠咽

周榮
胷鄉
天谿
食竇
腹哀

大包

大橫
腹結
府舍

箕門

血海

陰陵泉
地機
漏谷
三陰交
商丘
太白
太都

公孫

隱白

6. ARM GREATER YANG

SMALL INTESTINE MERIDIAN (手太陽小腸經)

Arm Greater Yang Small Intestine Meridian arises from the little finger and goes up through its ulnar side, along the back of the arm to the back of the shoulder. It then goes through the scapula to pass the neck and face into the eye.

It is related to the small intestines. Regulating *Arm Greater Yang Small Intestine Meridian* and its main acupuncture points are good for healing and preventing headache, giddiness, visual deterioration, watery eyes, deaf, face puffiness, backache, neurasthenia etc.

ARM GREATER YANG SMALL INTESTINE MERIDIAN

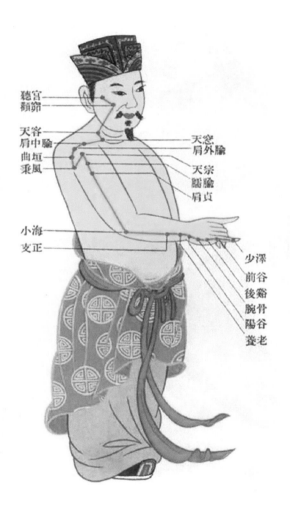

LEG GREATER YANG BLADDER MERIDIAN

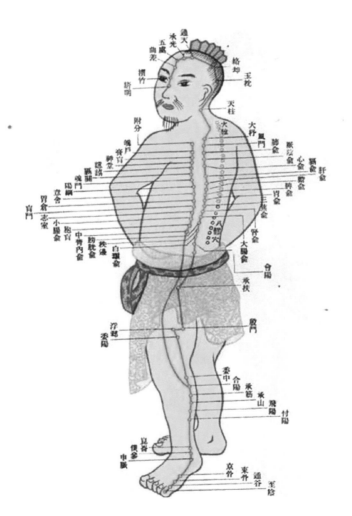

7. LEG GREATER YANG BLADDER MERIDIAN

(足太陽膀胱經)

Leg Greater Yang Bladder Meridian arises from the eye and goes up to the top of the head, then it goes down through the neck, the back and passes to the back of the leg and to the tip of the little toe.

It is related to the cerebral cortex, bladder and urinary system. Regulating *Leg Greater Yang Bladder Meridian* and its main acupuncture points are good for healing and preventing epilepsy, insomnia, giddiness, headache, Cardiovascular disease, sequelae (abnormal condition from previous disease), lower belly distension, painful urination and frequent urination etc.

LEG LESSER YIN KIDNEY MERIDIAN

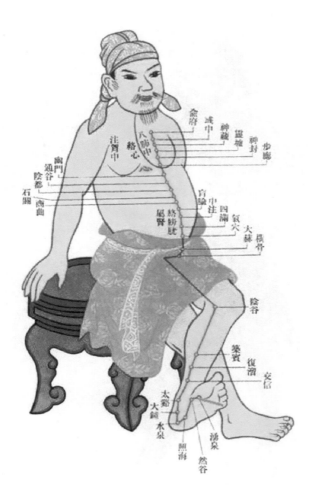

8. *LEG LESSER YIN KIDNEY MERIDIAN* (足少陰腎經)

The Leg Lesser Yin Kidney Meridian arises from under the little toe, crosses the foot arch to go up through the inside of the ankle and the leg into the chest.

It is related to kidney, reproductive system and urinary system. Regulating the *Leg Lesser Yin Kidney Meridian* and its main acupuncture points are good for healing and preventing bellyache, painful urination, frequent urination, impotence, premature ejaculation, myopia, menstrual colic and irregular menstruation

9. ARM ABSOLUTE YIN PERICARDIUM MERIDIAN

(手厥陰心包經)

Arm Absolute Yin Pericardium Meridian arises from the chest and goes through the inside of the arm to the tip of the middle finger. It is consequential to the pericardium and related to the health of the heart, chest and ribs.

Regulating *Leg Greater Yin Spleen Meridian* and its main acupuncture points are good for healing and preventing palpitation, chest congestion, painful swelling in the ribs, armpits, dry mouth and breast disease.

ARM ABSOLUTE YIN PERICARDIUM MERIDIAN

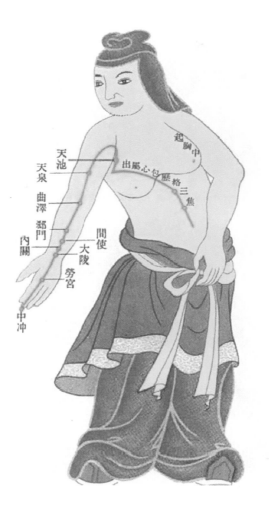

ARM LESSER YANG TRIPLE BURNER MERIDIAN

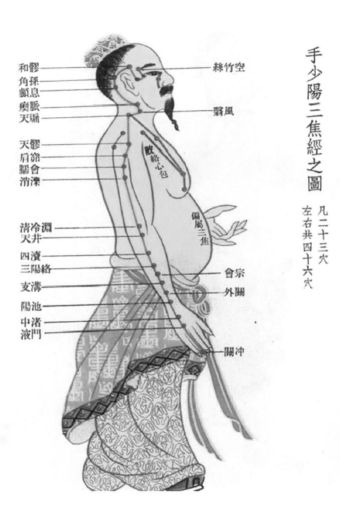

10. ARM LESSER YANG TRIPLE BURNER MERIDIAN

(手少陽三焦經)

Arm Lesser Yang Triple Burner Meridian arises from the ring finger and goes up through the median line of the outer side of the arm, the shoulder, the neck and the face to the eye.

The *Triple Burner Meridian* corresponds with organs which are related to the holistic health of the viscera (abdominal and other cavities). Regulating *Arm Lesser Yang Triple Burner Meridian* and its main acupuncture points are good for healing and preventing high blood pressure, stroke, migraine, eye redness, inflammation, deafness, tinnitus, insomnia, stiff neck, cold and the soft tissue injury of the upper limbs.

Triple Burner is the meridian that controls our fight, flight or freeze response. According Traditional Chinese Medicine (TCM), the triple burner impacts the immune system and our ability to manage stress.

There are many exercises involving the *Triple Burner Meridian* that may be used to reduce stress or to improve sleeping. For example: To calm worry or anxiety:

Place your flat hand on your heart and gently stroke the groove between and about an inch or so above the ring and little finger as shown page 84. Do this three times changing hands.

Rubbing and tracing the Triple Burner from the temple , around the ear, down shoulder and arm, back of hand and off the fourth (ring) finger may also be calming. Follow the red line on the drawing page 84.

85

11. LEG LESSER YANG GALLBLADDER MERIDIAN

(足少陽膽經)

Leg Lesser Yang Gallbladder Meridian arises from the outside corner of the eye. It then goes up at a frontal angle, then goes down behind the ear to pass through the neck.

The path then goes along the outer side of the chest and abdomen and moving down the leg all the way to pass the instep to the outer side of the forth toe.

Its corresponding organ is the gallbladder and it also related to the nervous system. Regulating *Leg Lesser Yang Gallbladder Meridian* and its main acupuncture points are good for healing and preventing dizziness, sciatica, abdominal distension and pain, jaundice and lower limbs numbness etc.

LEG LESSER YANG GALLBLADDER MERIDIAN

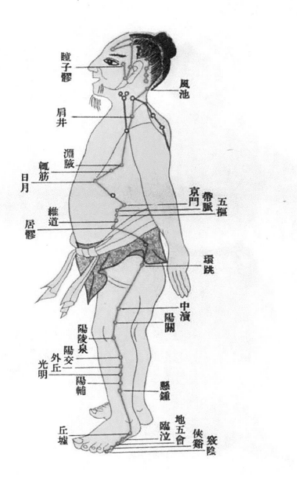

足少陽膽經之圖

凡四十三穴
左右共八十六穴

87

LEG ABSOLUTE YIN LIVER MERIDIAN

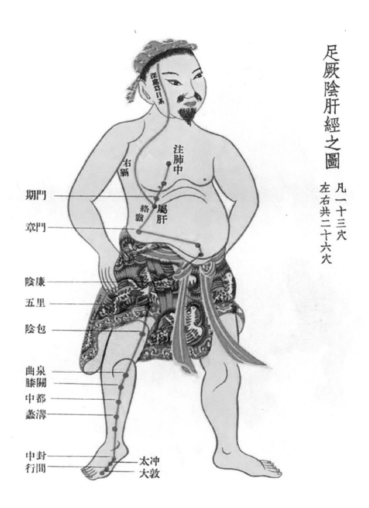

12. LEG ABSOLUTE YIN LIVER MERIDIAN (足厥陰肝經)

Leg Absolute Yin Liver Meridian arises from the big toe and passes through the instep. It then goes up through the median line of the inside of the leg, the abdomen and the chest all the way to the top of the head.

Its corresponding organ is the liver. Regulating *Leg Absolute Yin Liver Meridian* and its main acupuncture points are good for healing and preventing hepatitis, jaundice, soreness in the back, chest congestion, limb weakness, premature ejaculation and menstrual colic.

13. *REN MERIDIAN - CONCEPTION VESSEL* (任脉)

Ren Meridian - Conception Vessel arises from the lower belly, goes up through the center line of trunk to the jaw where it

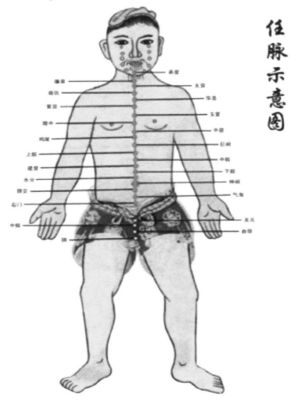

divides into two branches along the both sides of the nose up to the inferior orbit. *The Ren Meridian governs all the meridians of Yin*, Former Feminine Principle.

Regulating it and its main acupuncture points is good for healing and preventing impotence, premature ejaculation, nocturnal emission, menstrual colic, gastritis, abdominal distension, chest ache, chest congestion, convulsion, and vomiting.

14. DU MERIDIAN - GOVERNOR VESSEL (督脈)

Du Meridian - Governor Vessel arises from the lower belly to go down through the perineum and then goes up along the

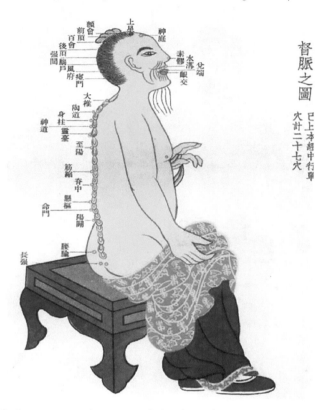

spine all the way to the top of the head - Bai Hui acupuncture point (百會穴). It governs all the meridians of Yang - Former Masculine Principle.

Regulating *Du Meridian* and its main acupuncture points are good for healing and preventing back problems, infant convulsion, headache, dizziness and the male disease such as kidney deficiency and impotence.

2. THE LOCATION METHOD FOR ACUPUNCTURE POINT

It is very important to find the relevant acupuncture points accurately before doing Self-massage. Generally, acupuncture points are located symmetrically on both sides of the body except for the acupuncture points which located on middle line of the torso, *Ren Meridian -Conception Vessel and Du Meridian - Governor Vessel.*

According to traditional Chinese acupuncture point locating method, our own fingers are the measurement for locating the acupuncture point by using the nose, eyes, ears, mouth, hair line, nipples, fingers and toes etc. as the reference (Figure 1).

It is so called *Finger Inch* (寸). For example, Guan Yuan acupuncture point (関元穴) is three Finger Inches (寸) which is about four fingers widths below the navel.

It should not be looked as a tiny point but a little spot when locating the acupuncture point. If there is a feel of sinking and a sense of sourness and numbness with little pain when pressing the acupuncture point, it means we have found the right place. To ensure accuracy, the person who receives the massage should use their own fingers to measure and find the position of the acupuncture point.

3. THE KEY POINTS OF SELF-MASSAGE

Press, squeeze, knead, pinch, rub(stroke) and push are the main methods of self-massage. The strength should be moderate when massaging certain parts of the body. It is not a simple friction just on the surface of the skin but a penetrable force with a downward pressure persistently. When you use the tip of your finger to knead or make circular motions on certain acupuncture point, it must keep sticking on this point which means the range of the circular motion should not be too big, otherwise your fingertip will deviate from the acupuncture point.

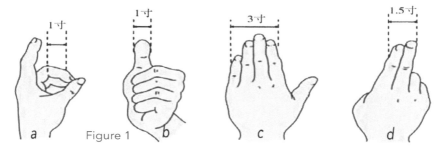

Figure 1

If your hand gets tied, have rest before beginning on the next massage item. You could also replace your fingertips with the knuckles to gain more power to stimulate the acupuncture point located in some strong muscles (Figure 2)
Not

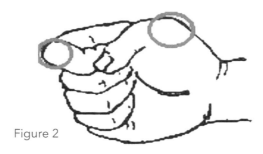

Figure 2

Notes:

CPSIA information can be obtained
at www.ICGtesting.com
Printed in the USA
LVHW071336020421
683316LV00001B/3